THE BARBARITY OF CIRCUMCISION AS A REMEDY FOR CONGENITAL ABNORMALITY

LECTOR HOUSE PUBLIC DOMAIN WORKS

THE BARBARITY OF CIRCUMCISION AS A REMEDY FOR CONGENITAL ABNORMALITY

HERBERT SNOW

ISBN: 978-93-90215-97-3

Published: 1890

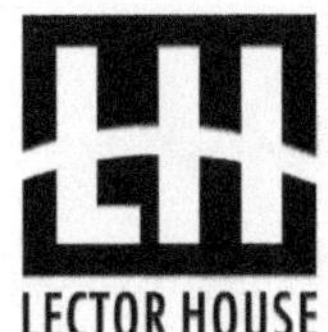

LECTOR HOUSE LLP
E-MAIL: lectorpublishing@gmail.com

THE BARBARITY OF CIRCUMCISION AS A REMEDY FOR CONGENITAL ABNORMALITY

BY

HERBERT SNOW, M.D. LOND. &C.

SURGEON TO THE CANCER HOSPITAL

1890

PREFATORY NOTE

To state that the object of this little work is to 'put down Circumcision' under the circumstances indicated, would, besides savouring of unpardonable arrogance, irresistibly suggest analogy to the example of a too famous alderman, who was determined to 'put down Suicide.'

If, however, the facts and arguments therein set forth contribute in some small measure towards the abolition of an antiquated practice involving the infliction of very considerable suffering upon helpless infants; and sanctioned, on extremely questionable grounds, by men of eminent authority; the following pages will not have been written in vain.

> More evil is wrought by want of thought,
> Than comes from want of heart.

Gloucester Place, Portman Square:
October 1800.

CONTENTS

Page

PREFATORY NOTE v

I. CIRCUMCISION AS A RELIGIOUS RITE. 1

II. NATURE OF CONGENITAL PHIMOSIS—PHYSIOLOGICAL IMPORTANCE OF THE PREPUCE.. 7

III. DANGERS AND RESULTS OF CONGENITAL PHIMOSIS—ACQUIRED PHIMOSIS. 10

IV. CUTTING OPERATIONS FOR THE RELIEF OF CONGENITAL PHIMOSIS; THEIR SUPPOSED ADVANTAGES. 12

V. DISADVANTAGES AND DANGERS OF CIRCUMCISION.. 19

VI. ABSENCE OF NECESSITY FOR CIRCUMCISION IN CASES OF CONGENITAL PHIMOSIS—THE RATIONAL TREATMENT OF THE LATTER. 23

VII. SUMMARY. 29

BIBLIOGRAPHY. 32

THE BARBARITY OF CIRCUMCISION AS A REMEDY FOR CONGENITAL ABNORMALITY

I.

CIRCUMCISION AS A RELIGIOUS RITE.

The earliest historical or quasi-historical notice of circumcision is to be found in Genesis xvii.; where Jahve enjoins upon Abraham the personal performance of this mutilation, as a sign of the covenant henceforward to subsist between them. Abraham, his son Ishmael, and all his male slaves forthwith underwent the prescribed operation; which thence-forward remained obligatory upon their posterity, though not without transient periods of desuetude. It was suffered to lapse during the passage of the Israelites through the wilderness, and was subsequently revived by Joshua (v. 5); again in the reign of Antiochus Epiphanes, when some of the Jews seem to have submitted to a plastic operation in order to obliterate its effects.[1]

The compulsory performance of circumcision was re-enacted for the last time by Mattathias, in the age of the Maccabees; and the law to this effect has remained in force until the present day.[2]

The terms in which the Deity addresses his commands to Abraham presuppose an already existing familiarity with the ritual ceremony on the part of the latter. Accordingly we find that it previously prevailed among the Colchians, Æthiopians, and ancient Egyptians of both the Upper and Lower Provinces (Gardner Wilkinson). Among the latter it appears to have become restricted, by the dawn of the historical period, to the priestly caste, and to those who desired initiation into the sacred mysteries. In the temple of Chunsu at Karnak is a delineation of the rite as performed on two young children, probably sons of Rameses II., the founder

---

[1] An account of the operation (seemingly then not infrequently resorted to) performed at a much later date for the above purpose, is to be found in *Celsus*, lib. vii. cap. xxv.

[2] According to Keating's *Cyclopædia of the Diseases of Children*, 1890, vol. iii., some of the rabbins now omit it; "in the teeth of a strong and growing popular prejudice." I am informed, however, by the Rev. S. Singer, to whom I am greatly indebted for a courteous reply to inquiry on the subject, that these congregations would not be regarded as orthodox; and that the innovation is unknown in the Old World.

of the building. It was apparently connected with the worship of Ra, the Sun God; and a seeming allusion to it in this connection is to be found in chapter xvii. of the 'Book of the Dead.' Notices of circumcision also appear in ancient Phœnician mythology.

There can be no question of its very great antiquity, or of its wide prevalence among ancient nations. Traditional descent from a primæval Stone Age is betrayed by casual notices in Holy Writ. Thus, in Exodus iv. 25, a sharp stone is the instrument of mutilation; and in Joshua v. 2, the marginal rendering is 'knives of flints.'[3]

The Hivites, the Canaanites (Phœnician), and many if not most of the nations with whom the Israelites were brought into contact after settlement in the Promised Land, appear to have practised circumcision at some period in their history. In the Old Testament we accordingly find the designation of 'the uncircumcised' specially reserved for the Philistines, and applied to these as a term of opprobrium.

The list of peoples by whom the circumcision of males has been, or is still, an established custom is sufficiently long. Among such races at the present day, 'an almost unbroken line may be traced from China to the Cape of Good Hope,' and unless perhaps in Europe (where comparatively slight traces of aboriginal manners and customs survive), we find the ceremony characteristic not only of savage tribes, but of nations ranking fairly high in the scale of civilisation; for instance, the Mexicans, and the ancient Aztec races of Central America. The Teanas and Manaos on the Amazon; the Salivos, Guamos, Otamocos, on the Orinoco; the negroes of the Congo, with many other tribes on both the west and east coasts of Africa, notably the Kaffirs, Bechuanas, and Hottentots; the Abyssinians (Christian), Nubians and modern Egyptians; the natives of Madagascar; most of the Australian aborigines; the Papuans, New Caledonians, inhabitants of the New Hebrides, of Java, of the Philippines, and of Fiji, are only a few that may be indicated. An approximation to the rite in the form of a slitting up of the prepuce was noticed among the Friendly Islanders by Captain Cook. Although not enjoined in the Koran, it is a universal practice among the Mohammedans, as a tradition from the ante-Mohammedan period.

A cognate operation upon *females* obtains among the modern Egyptians, the Nubians, the Abyssinians, as well as in many other parts of Africa among the negro races; also among the Malays on the shores of the Persian Gulf (Carsten Niebuhr), and on the banks of the Orinoco. As an ancient custom in Arabia and Egypt, it is noticed by Strabo.

Local variations of detail are found; as in the case of the Friendly Islanders just cited; and of the Madagascarians, who cut the flesh at three several times; the excised prepuce being eventually *swallowed* by some relative or other.

The date at which circumcision is performed varies considerably. Among the Jews, the eighth day is, of course, the selected period; probably from consideration

---

[3] In the *Lancet* of April 20, 1889, is figured a curious circumcising Instrument used by the Malays, who perform the rite upon boys at the age of eight years; and also upon females, about ⅛th inch being nipped off the extremity of the clitoris. In the ceremony performed on female children, variations exist; other tribes remove the nymphæ.

for the sacred number seven, for the seven days of uncleanness prescribed for the parturient mother (Lev. xii. 2), and for an idea that with the second cycle of seven days the infant then properly commenced its earthly life. Among the Arabs, it is deferred till the thirteenth year; the age at which their reputed ancestor, Ishmael, was submitted to it. And every race seems to have selected for itself what was considered the most suitable time. The Turks, for example, have chosen the seventh or eighth year; the Persians circumcise boys at thirteen, girls, between the ninth and the fifteenth year; and so on.

It is thus evident, not only that the rite is extremely ancient, but that it is impossible to refer the practice of circumcision to any single source; or to doubt that it originally arose among many widely-sundered peoples, as the result of a certain stage in man's mental evolution. The once widely-spread custom of the COUVADE, and other strange aboriginal practices, afford an illustrative analogy.[4]

Herodotus seems to have been the author, or at least the introducer, of the cleanliness theory; according to which the ceremony was invented from motives of hygiene. Philo Judæus ascribes the custom to four causes: 1. Cleanliness; 2. The avoidance of carbuncle (Qu. cancer?); 3. The symbolisation of purity of heart; 4. The attainment of numerous offspring.

Of these, it need hardly be said that the last has no foundation in fact; and the two preceding require no remark. The idea, however, that circumcision was initiated for purposes of cleanliness has lasted to the present day, and still appears to have considerable currency. Whatever may have been the social condition of the ancient Egyptians and Arabians, on behalf of both which races, as having been the source whence Abraham derived his evident familiarity with the custom, plausible pretensions have been put forth; it is simply preposterous to imagine for a moment that the numerous savage tribes (witness the Hottentots and the Australian aborigines) who practise it, could ever have been actuated by any such considerations. Its world-wide diffusion, again, totally forbids the supposition, either of its introduction into these tribes by contact with other nations more highly civilised; or of its adoption, by the former, while in a higher stage of sociology, from which they have subsequently become degraded. And this explanation is put finally out of court by the phenomenon of an analogous rite applied in sufficiently numerous quarters to the persons of females. In order, therefore, plausibly to account for the general prevalence of this strange mutilation, we are compelled to look elsewhere; and an examination of the religious ideas which are known to actuate primitive man, will afford a clue.

Copious illustrations of the working of such ideas among peoples emerging from barbarism can be traced in almost every page of the earlier books of our Old Testament; and, even in classical mythology, although overlaid by the later developments of a high civilisation, their influence is still not entirely effaced. The

---

[4] *La Couvade* was the designation of the unwritten law, according to which, directly an infant was brought into the world, the husband retired to bed and was sedulously nursed for a certain prescribed period; the mother, on the other hand, getting up and attending to the affairs of the household. Tylor speaks of it as "this once world-wide custom" (*Primitive Culture*, i. 76).

principle of substitution was familiar to all the nations of antiquity, to the Israelites not the least. Witness the universal resort to sacrifices, the theory of which is well indicated by that of Isaac in Genesis xxii. Further illustrative examples are afforded by the law of the scapegoat, in Leviticus xvi.; by the offering of children to Molech (Lev. xx. 2); and by the legend of Jephthah's daughter (Judg. xi.). With this, various ceremonies, involving either mutilation or the shedding of blood, were in vogue—for example, the priests of Baal (1 Kings xviii. 28); even cutting off the hair seems to have been in the nature of a representative sacrifice.[5]

Hence many German authorities cited in Keil's *Biblical Archæology* (vol. i. p. 415) consider circumcision as a relic of ancient sacrifice: the consecration of a part of the body for the whole. The different grades in the process of humanisation may be assumed to have been successively attained as follows. In the earliest periods, human sacrifice was probably universal; in the Bible, we have the episode of Jephthah's daughter, above referred to; and in the narrative of Abraham's purpose to offer Isaac there is not the slightest indication of surprise on the part of the patriarch when he received Jahve's commands; whence may be argued evident acquaintance with such deeds. Besides which, we hear of human sacrifice among the tribes contiguous to the Israelites, until a much later date. Even the Greeks and Romans occasionally resorted to this during the historical period; in the Homeric age, it appears to have been a not infrequent practice.

As, however, men progressed in culture and in humanity, such barbarity became impossible. Instead of putting their firstborn children (often by cruel methods, as in the sacrifices to Molech) to death, they propitiated the deity by an offer of the most precious member. Indeed, in the Genesis account of Abraham's circumcision, Mr. Moncure Conway considers (*Demonology and Devil Lore*, ii. 83) that the legend, subsequently obscured by later traditions, originally points to the performance of a much more severe operation. And when still more advanced, even this became impossible; the excision of a very small portion of the organ, not of indispensable necessity to the fulfilment of its functions, being substituted. After many generations had then passed over, the custom had become so firmly implanted in the mind and habits of the people, that its eradication was rendered a matter of extreme difficulty; even by new religious dispensations and more elevated modes of thought. Hence we find the rite among the Israelites made an exception to the fierce denunciation of mutilations in general, uttered by Jahve or by his messengers; and hence also, we see it (though not prescribed in the Koran) an ordinary modern custom throughout the whole of Islam, as well as among the Christian Abyssinians.

The practice of self-emasculation in honour of a divinity was a common feature in the worship of Chronos, of Cybele, and doubtless of many other among the earlier recipients of religious adoration; it is referred to (and not in terms of reprobation) at Matthew xix. 12. It has descended to modern times—witness the fanatical sects in Russia; and even persons of high intellectual calibre (as, for instance, Origen) have submitted to it. What men regarded as honourable and meri-

---

[5] Examples of the substitution principle among various *modern* races are to be found in Tylor's *Primitive Culture*, vol. ii. p. 36 *et seq.*

torious in themselves, they would be not unlikely to impose also on their children. The existence of such ascetic practices among partially civilised nations must not be lost sight of in the present connection; as helping us to comprehend the mental religious attitude of primæval man.

There can be little question that here we find our correct explanation of the origin and wide prevalence of circumcision. We are, however, no longer permitted to regard this as a hygienic custom, but simply and solely as a relic of barbarism; dating from an immemorial antiquity, long anterior to the first historical records, and when man was little, if at all, removed from savagery. The venerable age of the prescriptive rite, as well as the various social and religious phases through which the peoples adopting it have since successively passed, have effectually spiritualised it and have shed around it a certain halo of sentimentalism; but should not be suffered to obscure the only rational conception of its primary significance.

The sacrificial character of the act among the Israelites was indicated by a former custom of placing a pot of dust in the room where the ceremony was to take place; that, as we read in the third chapter of Genesis, being the allotted food of the serpent. The practice seems to have continued down to a recent period, but now to have fallen into disuse.

We thus clearly see that, beside being the sign of the covenant with the tribal deity, there was also involved the idea of a propitiatory sacrifice to the awful evil demons. The most clear instance of circumcision as an act intended to conciliate an offended divinity, or malignant spirit, appears in the strange story of Zipporah at Exodus iv. 24; where the vicarious nature of the rite is also plainly set forth. There is no apparent reason for identifying the Lord ('Adonai'); who sought to slay Moses, with Jahve; from whom Moses had just parted upon excellent terms. And there can be little doubt that Samael, to whom the scapegoat was subsequently offered (Lev. xvi. 20), or some similar dread power of darkness, is here meant.[6]

If the writer is not greatly in error, an impression prevails in some quarters that *Moses* either instituted anew or effectually perpetuated the rite of circumcision among the Israelites; as a useful measure of sanitation. However deservedly high the reputation of the great Hebrew lawgiver as a sanitarian, he does not seem entitled to credit in this connection; and alludes but casually to the ceremony, as to an already well-established custom, among certain directions for the treatment of the parturient woman at Leviticus xxii. 3. There is plainly no question of hygiene here involved. Dr. Asher (*The Jewish Rite of Circumcision*) considers that CHASTITY was the main purpose aimed at in the Divine injunction to Abraham; but, for reasons subsequently adduced, such a theory will be seen to have no foundation in fact.[7]

As the present is not an antiquarian treatise, only a very cursory historic or

---

[6] The imposition of circumcision by the Jews upon vanquished enemies, as the Idumeans and Itureans (Josephus, *Antiq.* B. 13) sounds the like note; there could hardly be any question of proselytism. At an earlier date these people would have been ruthlessly massacred *en masse*, like the Amalekites (1 Sam. xv. 8); slaughtered in great part, like the Moabites (2 Sam. viii.); or sacrificed, like Agag (1 Sam. xv. 3), to the deity of the conquerors.

[7] According to the same writer, it is absolutely impossible to say, in any given case

ethnic account of ritual circumcision is here inserted; many other curious and interesting particulars may be found in the authorities cited at the end of this volume, as well as in the copious German literature on the same subject. All that has been attempted in the preceding pages is to exhibit the custom in its original character; and (in so far as the pretensions advanced upon its behalf as a surgical procedure are concerned), divested of the traditional sanctity which is possibly largely answerable for some of the views promulgated by medical authors; whereby the general habit and practice of the medical profession become also of necessity deeply tinged.[8]

---

among the Mohammedans, whether circumcision has been performed or not; for, as the muco-cutaneous membrane has not been divided, 'the soft elastic skin of the penis easily comes forward and re-covers the glans.' He states that the performance of that particular portion of the ceremony which consists in tearing and removing the membrane in question, completely distinguishes the Jews from all the other nations of the world who practise the operation as a religious rite.

[8] Two cases of interest in this connection may be here noticed. Dr. Levy, a Jew dentist of Stettin, states (*Medical Record*, May 3, 1890) that, like his father before him, he was born without a foreskin; further, that his four brothers, who died in childhood, were similarly circumstanced.

The late Dr. Asher (*op. cit.*), who must be considered a high authority in such a matter (so far at least as concerns his co-religionists), says: 'No part of the human body is subject to so many varieties and irregularities as the penis and foreskin.' He believes total absence of the prepuce to be extremely rare, and doubts whether such a phenomenon has ever occurred; but seems to regard a partial deficiency as nothing unusual. He states that in most, if not all, instances of supposed congenital absence of this structure, a small portion of the skin will be found prolonged to the glans across the intervening fossa; which morsel, however small, must be excised by the Mohel, with the usual formalities. A note informs us that, according to Jewish tradition, the following personages never had foreskins: Adam, Seth, Noah, Shem, Melchizedek, Jacob, Joseph, Job, Moses, Balaam, Samuel, David, Jeremiah, Zerubbabel.

The second case bears upon the very heterodox theory of maternal impressions, and is reported in the same periodical, of dates Nov. 3, 1888, and March 23, 1889. It is that of a child born accurately circumcised, seven months and twenty days after the like operation on his elder brother (presumably in presence of the mother, although this is not stated). The local appearances in the two children are affirmed by Dr. Harvey, of Illinois, to have been exactly alike; 'the congenital case even showing the marks of the sutures.'

Both of the above cases, together with Dr. Asher's experiences, may be respectfully commended to the notice of Professor Weismann.

II.

NATURE OF CONGENITAL PHIMOSIS—PHYSIO-LOGICAL IMPORTANCE OF THE PREPUCE.

The word 'phimosis' (φιμόω, I bind) signifies that condition of the penis in which the prepuce cannot be retracted beyond the *corona glandis*; and which may be either congenital or factitious.

The latter is a pathological phenomenon, the product of injury or of disease. To apply the term 'abnormal' to the former is, however, hardly permissible, except when the difficulties in retraction are permanent and extreme; when they cannot be overcome by judicious perseverance, and by careful manipulation in the early weeks of infant life. A certain amount of adhesion between the two contiguous surfaces of mucous membrane is almost constantly present at birth, as a continuation of the normal intra-uterine agglutination (Keating's *Cyclopædia of the Diseases of Children*, 1890, vol. iii.; article by Dr. De Forest Willard).

The radical defect in congenital phimosis is thus the adhesion or imperfect separation of two muco-cutaneous surfaces, normally developed in close contact. As a rule, these are so slightly connected that a very slight degree of force is sufficient to part them; but in a considerable minority of instances the defect eventually becomes permanent; with the natural growth of the organ more difficulty is experienced in procuring retraction; and various disagreeable, or even dangerous, symptoms are prone then to make their appearance.

The complaint, however, is simply one of degree. If the adhesions at the margin of the urethral meatus are so tight that they fail to be quickly separated by the stream of urine directed against them—the force of which necessarily varies in different infants—considerable impediment to micturition results; and, perhaps usefully, serves to direct early attention to the state of the parts. In rare cases, no opening at all into the urethra has been discoverable; and complete retention has necessarily ensued. Very often, however, nothing of this sort happens for several weeks, months, or even years; and the existence, or rather persistence, of the disability may not be noticed at all until adolescence of adult life. The majority of instances lie between these extremes; not seldom unpleasant symptoms begin to be observed when the boy is a few months old; but there is a wide range of variation.

The penile and preputial layers of mucous or quasi-mucous membrane being firmly adherent, and growth of the glans penis proceeding apace, certain consequences necessarily follow.

The prepuce being (in extreme cases) tightly fixed to the margins of the urethral orifice, the *meatus urinarius* still retains the same calibre as when birth took place, and becomes far too small for the needs of the rapidly growing child. A difficulty in effectually voiding the bladder is experienced, and may eventually result in complete retention. The little patient tugs at the seat of unpleasant sensation; and this elongates the folds of skin at the extremity of the penis, normally somewhat redundant, and extremely distensile. The muscular force of the bladder being spent upon overcoming the obstruction at the narrow meatus, the urine trickles out feebly, and 'balloons' in the soft pouches beyond, which continuously retain a few drops. Hence great local irritation and excoriation.

It is not warrantable, however, to speak of *contraction* of the penile mucous membrane. No contraction takes place, except as a consequence of inflammatory attacks; and these, in the infant, are rarely sufficient to cause any material shrinking. The phenomenon is simply one of natural development under a rigid restraining envelope; and though eventually the aperture is found narrow enough, the 'contraction' is relative only. So also, in every male child there is more or less seeming redundancy of skin at the end of the penis;—for natural physiological reasons. The condition is apt, as first stated, to become factitiously enhanced under the pressure of urinary obstruction. But there is seldom or never a *real superfluity of integument* in this locality *ab initio*; in excess of what the subsequent needs of the full-developed organism may be reasonably supposed to warrant. It is requisite to lay some stress on these two points, as tending materially to influence our conceptions of the practice condemned in this pamphlet.

Although plainly not absolutely essential to the due increase in bulk of the penis, or to the subsequent performance of its functions, it is *prima facie* obvious that the prepuce must be intended to subserve some useful purpose. That, according to Dr. Willard (Keating's *Cyclopædia*), 'is to protect the head of the organ, during the years when the penis is but a portion of the urinary apparatus; and later, by its friction over the sensitive corona, to enhance the ejaculatory orgasm.' The latter half of this statement may fairly be questioned, as the prepuce is completely retracted during coition; and so no friction over 'the corona' can well take place under ordinary conditions. The first part, however, is unimpugnable; and to it may be added some consideration of the protection afforded during the first efforts at functional use.

Some measure of the degree in which the glans penis is shielded from external irritating agencies is afforded by the sensations of the adult for the first time deprived of this appendage; or in whom the latter is kept retracted for any length of time, contrary to preceding habit. Extreme discomfort, indeed considerable soreness and actual pain, are complained of; until tolerance becomes established, and until the delicate membrane has by exposure and friction become so hardened that the absence of its former covering is no longer noticed, a period occupying commonly several weeks.[9]

---

[9] The fact that many adults, of not too sensitive organisation, gradually acquire a habit of retaining the foreskin partially or even entirely retracted, is of course not lost sight of. But this in no way affects the question of its *sudden* removal, or of the protection afforded

In the case of young children, the unpleasant sensations involved must be relatively far greater; considering their physical helplessness and their more impressionable nervous system.

According, moreover, to the authority previously cited, early removal of the prepuce is apt to be followed by *progressive sclerosis*, with attendant evils of *contracted meatus, balanitis*, &c. And, failing this, 'the exposure of the tender skin to the friction of the clothing, &c. tends to keep up a state of abnormal excitement during the early years of life.'

It thus becomes apparent that, apart from any risks involved by operative procedures, ablation of the prepuce, whether in infant or in adult, is not a measure to be undertaken lightly, or without satisfactory evidence of positive necessity.

by the structure in question to infants of tender years.

III.

DANGERS AND RESULTS OF CONGENITAL PHIMOSIS—ACQUIRED PHIMOSIS.

A perfectly healthy condition of the male generative organs is compatible only with perfect mobility of the prepuce over the gland which it envelopes. So, in the absence of this, we encounter a number of ill consequences, some local only; some affecting the well-being, and even the life, of the entire organism.

The parts being extremely vascular, and in very intimate relation with the central nervous system; we very naturally find that congenital phimosis, interfering with the normal growth of the glans penis, is prone to develop various reflex neurotic disorders or diseases; of which some have been minutely described by Dr. Sayre.[10] Thus forms of *paralysis* may ensue; either confined to a single group of muscles, and simulating club-foot, or of a more general character. *Epilepsy, reflex cough, convulsions, choreic movements of the limbs,* are extreme examples; but a milder instance of the same causes in operation shows itself in young infants, as *nocturnal restlessness with defective nutrition. Hip-joint disease* and *spinal caries* may be simulated, and the mal-assimilation of food may eventually produce such gross deformities as *bowing of the legs.* Chronic *priapism* is a not uncommon occurrence.

Obstruction to the free discharge of urine may produce symptoms of severe *vesical irritation,* occasionally supposed to indicate stone in the bladder. The straining efforts at micturition may cause *hernia* or *prolapse of the rectum;* the *nocturnal incontinence* of children is not unfrequently traceable to the same source. *Epistaxis* has been described. Retention of urine in the folds of the elongated foreskin, together with the child's habit of pulling this, induce a condition of soreness which causes great smarting whenever micturition takes place, and induces the patient to defer that act as long as possible. Hence may in time result *dilatation of the bladder, cystic kidneys, and death.* Even *eczema* of the abdominal wall has been thus produced; and has disappeared when the cause was removed, as in a case cited by Dr. Hayes Agnew (*Principles of Surgery,* 1881).

When the patient is allowed to reach adult life with the disability unrelieved, he becomes subject to attacks of *balanitis;* and the parts may ulcerate or even slough. In a case seen by the writer, where at the time no symptoms of inflammation were present, the retained deposits of smegma had ulcerated through the prepuce at various points—projecting from this exactly like chalk-stones from the fingers of a gouty person. In a unique case cited by Erichsen, 'Dr. Wisham, of Fyzabad, re-

---

[10] *Orthopædic Surgery,* p. 14. See also Hilton, *Rest and Pain,* p. 276.

moved no fewer than 426 calculi, varying in size from a pin's head to a small bean, from this situation, in the person of a native of India, sixty years of age, who came under treatment for what appeared to be a large tumour at the end of the penis, the true nature of which was not detected until, on removing it, the knife grated against the contained calculi.' The defect constitutes a serious impediment to impregnation; in the event of an acquired local disorder, its presence seriously hinders diagnosis, and altogether precludes appropriate treatment. It has been supposed, and not without plausibility, to predispose to *epithelioma*. A case is given by Mr. Oliver Pemberton; and others have been reported. There can be no question that, under such circumstances, the presence of malignant disease about the glans would much longer remain undetected than in a normal state of the parts; and that the prospects of cure by operative removal would be proportionately lessened. Only comparatively mild examples of phimosis, in which the adhesions produced little or no constriction, and did not at all interfere with urination, could thus have been suffered to pass unrelieved until the subjects were far past maturity.

Phimosis, as an *acquired* condition, is of frequent occurrence in an *acute* form; as the result of inflammatory œdema of the prepuce in youths and adults. This, again, may be a consequence of simple balanitis, the result of want of cleanliness, combined with disordered general health and a catarrhal state of all the mucous membranes; in which event it usually yields to mild measures, such as the injection of warm fluids under the foreskin. In by far the greater number of instances it is produced by venereal infection; and imperatively needs prompt operation, usually in the guise of slitting up the structure on a director. In a *chronic* form, slowly and gradually coming on, and very intractable to remedial measures, it is not seldom seen in old men of gouty habit; and of consequently unhealthy and irritable mucous membranes.

The pathology and treatment of ACQUIRED phimosis do not fall within the scope of the present work, but it is necessary to point out that these are essentially different from those of the congenital; and that the latter needs consideration upon principles totally diverse.

In the congenital we have to deal with tissues *perfectly healthy*, and with skin peculiarly elastic and distensile. In the factitious, all the parts are more or less altered by *disease*, acute or chronic; and as a sequel to the latter, or to repeated attacks of the former, *true contraction* takes place; the prepuce often attaining a hard and gristly consistence, under which condition simple dilatation is difficult or impossible. The phenomenon is rarely, if ever, seen in association with congenital phimosis; barring gout or venereal taint in addition.

NOTE.—The infrequency of *cancerous disease* attacking the penis, renders it unsafe to dogmatise upon any supposed causal relationship between that malady and the presence or absence of the foreskin, and does not appear to warrant any stronger assertion on this point than that which is recorded on the previous page.

IV.

CUTTING OPERATIONS FOR THE RELIEF OF CONGENITAL PHIMOSIS; THEIR SUPPOSED ADVANTAGES.

From the preceding, the evils or dangers incurred by permitting a male child to reach adult life; or, in the event of pressing symptoms, to pass even a few weeks or months with this disability unrelieved; are sufficiently obvious. Although, as Dr. Willard (*op. cit.*) states, the adhesions between prepuce and glans can nearly always be broken down with sufficient readiness during the first few weeks after birth, there can be little doubt that, without conspicuous necessity, the medical practitioner will seldom care to 'make the baby cry,' and thus draw down upon himself vigorous maternal reproaches. It seems, moreover, hardly judicious to encourage any tampering by nurses or midwives, probably more or less ignorant and unskilled. We may take it for granted, therefore, that nothing will usually be done until the child is several months old; when some more energetic treatment will be requisite to remedy the condition in question. In milder cases no notice will probably be taken of the abnormality for at least several years, and its presence may be detected only by accident; the adhesions in such are trivial, and do not interfere with normal growth; hence are, as a rule, easily overcome.[11]

Although less severe measures have been from time to time brought forward and advocated, the operation of circumcision is, to all intents and purposes, the only procedure in general use for remedying congenital phimosis; and as the latter is very common, so also is the performance of this ancient sacrificial rite among that large majority of the population who are otherwise in no way committed to it. There is a simplicity and thoroughness about the little amputation which may perhaps commend it to the surgical mind; and there are unquestionably certain superficial advantages of a hygienic nature about the patient's subsequent condition; though it may be doubted whether these are by any means so considerable as has been made to appear.

However this may be, it goes without saying that no other curative proceeding has so far met with any wide favour in the medical profession; and, if one may judge from their published opinions, the leading exponents of medical practice

[11] In Druitt's *Surgeon's Vade-Mecum*, 9th edition, p. 662, are the notes of a case of 'congenital phimosis of the tightest kind' in an adult of twenty-three. Circumcision was threatened; but the affection readily yielded to the injection of warm water daily. There are probably many similar.

and opinion, in this country at least, are so pleased with circumcision and its results that they would willingly see the Mosaic Laws in this particular extended to the whole Christian population, whether affected by phimosis or not. Witness Mr. Jonathan Hutchinson:

> It is surely not needful to seek any recondite motive for the origin of the practice of circumcision. No one who has seen the superior cleanliness of a Hebrew penis can have avoided a very strong impression in favour of the removal of the foreskin. It constitutes a harbour for filth, and is a constant source of irritation. It conduces to masturbation, and adds to the difficulties of sexual continence. It increases the risk of syphilis in early life, and of cancer in the aged. I have never seen cancer of the penis in a Jew, and chancres are rare.—*Archives of Surgery.*

Arguments by this distinguished surgeon, in favour of extension of the custom as a matter of ordinary routine to every male Gentile, are to be found in the *Medical Times and Gazette*, December 1, 1855; together with a reference to previous utterances in an identical sense.

Erichsen (*Surgery*, Ninth Edition, 1888, vol. ii. p. 1188) says:

> Every child who has a congenital phimosis ought to be circumcised; and even those who, without having phimosis, have an abnormally long and lax prepuce, would be improved greatly in cleanliness, health, and morals by being subjected to the same operation. It would be well if the custom of Eastern nations, whether it be regarded as a religious rite or only as a time-honoured observance, were introduced amongst us.

In Holmes's *System of Surgery*, 1883, we read:

> Circumcision is the operation required in children; and it is best adapted for adults also when the skin is redundant, and the margins of the preputial opening are thickened.

Mr. W. H. Jacobson (*Operations of Surgery*, 1889) says:

> This operation is still not practised often enough, especially among poorer patients; amongst whom many practitioners still treat phimosis as a matter of but little importance.

Some of the pretensions set forth above on behalf of circumcision will be subsequently referred to; but on the plea for a general extension of the rite to nations not impelled thereto by special Divine command, it may be remarked that several Jewish surgeons who have written upon the topic by no means regard this with an eye of favour; and have, in fact, gone even so far as to denounce in the strongest terms its compulsory performance among their co-religionists.[12]

---

[12] Dr. Asher (*op. cit.*) does not disapprove of circumcision, but his evidently strong religious bias, and the fact that his whole work is composed from an ecclesiastical point of view, with the express sanction and co-operation of ecclesiastical dignitaries, constitutes him a far from independent (negative) witness.

For their dislike, they advance what appear to be very adequate reasons; and, in such a matter they must have enjoyed a far wider special experience than any practitioner without the Hebrew pale.

The following extract from Erichsen's *Science and Art of Surgery* (Ninth Edition, 1888) may be regarded as a typical account of the ordinary surgical operation in vogue at the present day. The italics are the present writer's:

> Circumcision in boys or adults may be most conveniently performed in the following way. The surgeon restrains hæmorrhage during the operation by tying a tape tightly around the root of the penis, or by compressing the organ in Clover's circumcision tourniquet, a most useful instrument, which can be slackened or tightened at any time. He next draws the elongated prepuce slightly forwards, until the portion of it which corresponds to the back of the glans is brought just in front of that structure. He then seizes the projecting prepuce immediately in front of the glans with a pair of narrow-bladed polypus-forceps, which he gives to an assistant, who must hold them tightly; or he grasps it and protects the glans by means of a plate which I have had constructed for this purpose. With one sweep of the bistoury he cuts off all that portion of the integument which projects beyond the forceps, which are then taken away. It will now be found that he has removed only a circle of skin, but that the mucous membrane lining it still tightly embraces the glans; this he slits up, by introducing the point of a pair of scissors at the preputial orifice; and then, trimming off the angles of the flaps, he turns back the mucous membrane and attaches it to the edge of the cutaneous incision by a sufficient number of fine catgut sutures. Before introducing these, he will generally find it necessary *to ligature a small artery on each side of the penis, and one or two in the frænum.* The best dressing in children will be some simple ointment, such as boracic acid ointment, or the glans may be simply smeared with a little vaseline. After every act of micturition the parts should be well sponged with boracic acid lotion or Condy's fluid and water. In the adult, union by first intention may often be obtained by a dry dressing of iodoform-wool thickly covered with collodion, so as to protect it from the urine. This may be left unchanged for four or five days. *There is usually a good deal of swelling of the mucous membrane about the frænum, and some solid œdema usually remains for some weeks after the operation.* This gradually subsides, and a linear cicatrix remains, which causes the patient no inconvenience....
>
> *The chief points to be attended to in the performance of this operation, and on which its after-success is most dependent, are*—1. That too much skin be not removed; 2. That the mucous membrane be slit up to the base of the glans; 3. That too much of it be not removed; 4. That all bleeding vessels be tied with catgut ligatures, which

must be cut short; 5. That the mucous membrane be well turned back, so as to cover the gap left by the retracted skin; 6. That all sutures be of catgut, which will be absorbed, and thus save the pain of taking them out.

The *modus operandi* of different surgeons varies in particular details, usually of a slight and unimportant character. The pithy description contained in Maunders *Operative Surgery* may be appropriately quoted:

> The extremity of the foreskin being seized with forceps is drawn well forwards; the whole prepuce is embraced with the blades of dressing-forceps, immediately anterior to the *glans penis*, and cut off in front of the latter instrument. As soon as the forceps are removed, the skin will become retracted, leaving the mucous membrane still about the glans; this is slit up longitudinally as far as the corona, when it may be turned back, and its edge will come into apposition with the circular wound in the skin. The operation is now complete; but in the adult it will be well to introduce a few interrupted sutures.

The prepuce has sometimes been *slit up longitudinally on a director*. Although well suited to cases of adventitious phimosis in the adult, the method is in no way adapted to the congenital form, and has never found general favour with the medical profession. It has no advantages over circumcision; although retaining the prepuce, it still leaves the glans largely uncovered; and the sharp corners of the divided skin, unless trimmed and rounded off, produce a very unsightly after-appearance.

In performing circumcision many surgeons hold the clamp or dressing forceps which protect the glans inclined obliquely downwards and forwards, so as to leave a portion of the prepuce in the neighbourhood of the frænum unremoved. As one of the main advantages claimed for the operation is the prevention of future infection by retention of morbid material in the preputial folds, such a practice would seem to indicate a lurking disbelief in the validity of this pretension. If it be reasonable and right to excise the structure on these grounds, and if that proceeding be attended by such salutary effects; it is only logical not to do things by halves, but to make the excision as complete as possible. Thus Liston made his section near the frænum, 'so as to retain the skin on the glans, which is of advantage.' The use of the *elastic ligature*, and of the *écraseurs*, both ordinary and galvanic, for the performance of circumcision, are cruel and fantastic modes of effecting that object, which hardly need any expression of condemnation; and which it is difficult to believe can ever have been seriously advocated. Keyes (*Diseases of the Urinary Organs*, 1888), after breaking up adhesions with an oiled probe, marks an aniline line around the foreskin, and amputates the skin, &c., in front of this mark; thus previously estimating the amount of tissue to be removed.[13]

---

[13] An immense variety of operative procedures for phimosis, or even of details in the performance of ordinary circumcision, might be quoted. *Quot homines, tot operationes.* Their multiplicity, and the very contradictory nature of the advantages claimed for each, strongly indicate that neither the results of slitting operations, nor those of entire or partial

For operations involving the amputation of the whole, or nearly the whole prepuce, the following advantages are claimed:—

(*a*) Greatly enhanced local cleanliness throughout after-life.

(*b*) Greater chastity; and the preclusion of immoral personal habits.

(*c*) A smaller liability to venereal contagion in after-life.

(*d*) A diminished proneness to eventual cancerous disease.

In respect of the first of these it may be conceded that, among a people naturally of uncleanly habits, abstraction of the prepuce would at any rate prevent mischief resulting from compulsory retention of the smegma. Whether it would lead to more frequent ablutions is perhaps doubtful; as also whether the plea has any valid efficacy in regard of persons belonging to the better classes, or to nations not specially distinguished (like the Oriental) for their disregard of the most elementary laws of personal hygiene. With savage tribes or with such races as the Chinese (many of whom are said to be completely washed from head to foot on two occasions only—when they enter the world, and when they have quitted it), anything conducing to more complete bodily cleanliness in after-life is certainly worthy of consideration; and probably of approval, even when it necessitates a surgical operation. But to apply this reasoning to more civilised peoples seems hardly warrantable on the facts in view. Shaving the head, or plucking out the nails would materially conduce to subsequent freedom from dirt; but no one would seriously advocate either of these as habitual customs; and the practice under discussion in no way differs from them, so far as the principle involved is concerned.

The second of the reasons above assigned is one which has probably great weight in determining the practice of many surgeons; and it has even been gravely contended by one of the Jewish communion that the Deity instituted the rite among the Israelites in order to promote their greater purity and continence.[14]

This suggests the irrepressible commentary that, whatever the case in bygone years, the operation seems now to have wholly lost its salutary effects in the direction indicated, as Mr. Jonathan Hutchinson (*Medical Times and Gazette, loc. cit.*) himself testifies.

---

excision of the prepuce, are found uniformly satisfactory. Thus, in addition to the methods described in the text, it may be noted that Jobert de Lamballe and others divide the foreskin on both sides of the frænum without excision; Van Buren makes two cuts, one on the dorsum and one near the frænum, subsequently removing the two flaps; Dr. R. W. Taylor (*American Journal of Syphilis and Dermatology*, October, 1872) makes two *lateral* incisions with scissors. While, as above stated, some surgeons prefer to hold the forceps which guard the glans obliquely, from above downwards and forwards, so as to leave a certain portion of the skin about the frænum; Mr. Howse (*Guy's Hospital Reports*) advocates the careful removal of the frænum, in order to prevent subsequent œdema. Simple incision on a director was formerly preferred by many, though for congenital phimosis it has now probably fallen into disuse. In contrast with the careful devices for retaining part of the prepuce, or for ensuring that too much be not cut away, Sir W. Fergusson and Professor Humphrey find it best to amputate the structure as radically as possible. On this point see cases by Mr. Reginald Harrison, referred to at page 20.

[14] See the *Lancet*, December 12, 1874. Dr. Asher (*op. cit.*) also takes the same view.

Doubtless anything which might tend to enhance the chastity of many modern nations would be well worthy of serious consideration; with a view to its universal adoption. Strange to say, however, certain of those medical men who have investigated the question with opportunities of special experience, largely base their opposition to the practice of ritual circumcision upon the ground that removal of the foreskin in early life leads to premature sexual excitement, and a corresponding disposition to onanism. (Levit, *Allg. Wiener med. Zeit.*, November 17, 1874.)

In the *Lancet* of April 4, 1869, two cases materially bearing upon this point are reported. One is that of a Jew, aged thirty-five, suffering from 'spinal paralysis,' which he attributed to a habit of persistent masturbation in childhood or youth. And allusion is made to a younger brother of the same patient; who, as a consequence of the same, had acquired spermatorrhœa, Dr. Willard (Keating's *Cyclopædia*) says:

> I have failed to find any statistics proving that the circumcised masturbate less frequently, or are more virtuous than others; and the exposure of the tender skin to friction of clothing &c., tends to keep up a state of abnormal excitement during the early years of life.

'Where doctors differ, who shall decide?' And in face, therefore, of such directly contradictory opinions from professional witnesses, it is difficult to believe that ablation of the prepuce is of material avail, either in precluding masturbation, or in promoting the subsequent chastity of the adult individual.

On the third of the reasons assigned for advocating circumcision—the prevention of venereal disease when manhood is attained—Mr. Jonathan Hutchinson, whose testimony cannot but receive considerable weight, remarks that chancres are rare in the Jew. The observation has not been controverted; but must be received with a certain amount of hesitancy, in consequence of an evident bias in favour of radical measures of operative treatment. It seems rather to need confirmation by surgeons of the Jewish race, practising especially among their co-religionists. The present writer has been unable to discover any evidence in support from such a quarter. The authority last cited points out that cicatricial tissue is of all others least resistent to infection; and in the writer's own confessedly few opportunities for research in this particular field the number of Jews who have displayed remote but unmistakable indications of previous syphilitic taint has not appeared small. It is not improbable that a Hunterian sore developed upon scar-tissue, or upon the hardened integument of a denuded glans, would be far more trivial in character, more transient, less productive of inconvenience, and less easily recognisable, than the same in a normal state of the parts; the after-effects being, of course, identical. Such primary lesions in a people notoriously rather negligent of their person would seldom come under the notice of the medical practitioner. So, failing further evidence, the provisional verdict upon this question must be the Scotch one, 'Not proven.'

But even if the above assertion be accepted in respect of true syphilis, it assuredly fails to hold good with reference to other varieties of venereal disease.

Thus Mr. Jonathan Hutchinson's oft-quoted statistics[15] (*Medical Times and Gazette,* December 1, 1885), in his own words, 'prove that, though in proportion of nearly a third to the other patients, they (Jews) furnish nearly half the cases of gonorrhœa.'

The last-named motive for circumcision, although, in the passage quoted at the beginning of this section, it has been stamped with the approval of the same high authority, needs but transient allusion. It is *a priori* probable that congenital phimosis prolonged into adult life renders the subject thereof somewhat more likely to develop local malignant disease than any one not so circumstanced; the resulting attacks of inflammation and of unhealthy ulceration, &c., may be naturally expected to lead to the growth of papillomata, as well as to maintain a chronic condition of lowered vitality. But the comparative rarity of epithelioma in this particular locality would deprive the allegation, even if this were positively established as an indisputable fact, of any weight as an argument for the removal of the prepuce. Moreover, it is obviously a reason not for the routine performance of circumcision, but for the relief of phimosis; by whatever means attempted or proposed.

---

[15] The following is Mr. Hutchinson's statistical table derived from his practice at the Out-patient department of the Metropolitan Hospital:

Cases		Gonorrœa	Syphilis	Proportion of gonorrhœa to syphilis
Not Jews	272	107	165	0·6 to 1
Jews	58	47	11	4·3 to 1

On these figures a plausible inference might perhaps be founded, that what the Jew saves in immunity from syphilis he, to a certain extent, loses in increased proclivity to gonorrhœa; certainly the least of the two evils.

Mr. Hutchinson goes on to state that of 252 children under the age of five years, 27 out of 179 Christians exhibited symptoms of congenital syphilis in a well-marked form; while only 3 out of 73 Jews were thus affected, the proportion thus being 1 in 6 among the Christians, while only 1 in 24 among the Jews. Again, of 97 women (two-thirds being married), of whom 92 were Christians and 5 Jews, 61 of the former were syphilised; against a blank return among the latter. Upon the evidence of these statistics, Mr. Hutchinson advocates a general adoption of the rite of circumcision by Western nations!

Upon his own showing, however, the benefit to be derived from such a sweeping innovation, supposing that this were practicable, is not so very large; for 11 syphilised Jews out of a total of 58 with venereal disease, is a tolerably respectable proportion. The inferences here drawn, moreover, do not appear to have been confirmed by careful statistical observation carried out by other medical practitioners; among whom those of Jewish birth should be able to give specially valuable testimony. The field of inquiry was comparatively small; statistics drawn from the out-patient department of a general hospital are, for obvious reasons, not always of the most reliable character; and the conclusions may be vitiated by the facts suggested in the text. Hence, although they refer to but one venereal malady, it is hardly possible to acquiesce in them implicitly, even in this limited respect; without some confirmation drawn from a much more extended field of research.

V.

DISADVANTAGES AND DANGERS
OF CIRCUMCISION.

As a surgical operation, circumcision is commonly performed with so much impunity that many surgeons will probably not be disposed to admit the possibility of its being attended by any danger to life; and there can be no doubt that it is but seldom followed by a fatal result. Still, with any breach of surface whatever, there must be a chance of blood-poisoning and of the absorption of septic materials; and, in the case of a child liable to hæmophilia, it cannot be doubted that serious consequences might readily ensue.

Thus, in the third century it was enacted by the rabbins (*Talmud, Treatise Jebamoth*, 646) that, after two deaths in the same family from this cause, the ceremony was to be omitted; and the prohibition has continued in force ever since. Maimonides inculcates the utmost caution in the performance of the rite, and insists that 'in case of doubtful sickness, a child must not be circumcised; since danger to life overrides the whole ceremonial law.' (*Maimonides on Circumcision*, ch. i.). At the present date it is always effected by an expert (Mohel), who is not infrequently a qualified medical man; and accidents are guarded against with jealous care.[16]

The ancient plan, according to which the operator received in his mouth (previously filled with wine) the extremity of the lacerated member, is now wholly or in great part abolished among the Jewish community; it being found that both syphilis and tuberculosis were thus communicated to the infant.[17]

The *Lancet* of October 1, 1870, quotes from the *Wiener Med. Presse* the particulars of two cases, reported by Dr. Schwartz, of boys circumcised at the usual period; who subsequently died from phlegmonous inflammation and sloughing of the part, one five and the other twenty-five days subsequently to the operation. In the same periodical for December 5, 1874, may be found allusion to the experience of Dr. Kohn, himself a Jew; who stated at a medical society in Vienna, that during a practice of thirty-five years he had known six deaths from this source (*Allg. Wiener Med. Zeit.* November 17, 1874). He himself had thus lost a child of his own.

---

[16] The most scrupulous and minute precautions for obviating any danger to life are enjoined by the Talmud. The ceremony is not permitted to take place at all unless the child is in perfectly sound health; and that Mohel, whose conscience may convict him of having caused the death of an infant by his negligence, is forbidden ever to officiate again.

[17] A case of tuberculosis thus contracted is reported in the *British Medical Journal* of March 5, 1887; and twelve other instances are also mentioned in the same paragraph.

However such fatality may be attributed to the neglect of all hygienic rules among the poorer classes of Jews; it can hardly be doubted that, under even the most favourable conditions, septic poisoning or uncontrollable hæmorrhage *must* occasionally happen, albeit extremely rare; and this whether the operation has been performed from ritual or from surgical motives. To the absence of such cases reported in medical literature, too much weight must not be attributed.[18]

It is rather upon the minor consequences, immediate or subsequent, that those who object to the practice have founded their opposition; and of such there has been no lack, especially among medical men who have been themselves Jews, and who have thus necessarily enjoyed the fullest experience of its effects. Thus the *Lancet* of December 5, 1874, mentions a pamphlet by Dr. Levit, demonstrating the evils of the custom. He speaks of the premature beginning of sexual excitement in boys deprived of their prepuce, and the disposition to onanism so common to Eastern nations; he regards circumcision as a criminal manipulation; and calls upon the medical profession to oppose the practice, even at the risk of losing favour at the hands of the Jewish families they attend. And his arguments are effectually sustained by Dr. Kohn. Dr. Schwartz, in recording the fatal cases above quoted, 'deprecates the custom with great warmth, and expresses the wish that it may be laid aside.'

Mr. R. W. Parker (*British Medical Journal*, July 19, 1879) refers to a child (one of a family of bleeders) who, being circumcised, nearly bled to death. He also says: 'Diffuse cellulitis of the penis is not an uncommon complication after this operation in unhealthy, ill-fed, and badly-cared-for children.'

Dr. Mastin, in *Gaillard's Medical Journal*, speaks of the great frequency with which he has been consulted by Jews for chronic urethral discharges, irritable urethra, and other affections of the genito-urinary organs. He describes 'the preternaturally small meatus which results from early removal of the prepuce by circumcision.' (*Medical Record*, December 10, 1885.) Elsewhere in the same periodical (*Medical Record*, vol. xxi.) we are informed that 95 per cent. of young male Jew adults have this contracted meatus.

Shorn of its natural protective covering, the muco-cutaneous covering of the glans soon becomes true dermoid tissue. Mr. J. Hutchinson (*loc. cit.*) speaks of 'every one who is acquainted with the effects of circumcision in rendering the delicate mucous membrane of the glans hard and skin-like.' Contact with the clothing, &c., necessarily induces a chronic inflammatory condition of the part, followed commonly by contraction and condensation. We cannot with impunity rashly interfere with any of Nature's dispositions, however seemingly insignificant.

This hard skinlike condition of the integument upon the glans penis, with its concomitant of narrowed urethral aperture, may be regarded as the normal result of circumcision. In the hands of bungling operators, however, far worse consequences may follow. Thus J. Bell (*Manual of Operations in Surgery*, 1866) 'has known the glans penis included in the incision in *at least* one instance.' (The italics are his own.) Mr. Reginald Harrison (*Diseases of Urinary Organs*, 3rd Edition, 1887)

[18] The writer has been unable to discover any mortality statistics of ritual circumcision, and apparently none exist. Dr. Asher (*op. cit.*) makes a remark to the same effect.

has treated two *varieties* of urethral stricture after circumcision which have not turned out well; in two *cases*, the extremity of the glans penis, including the meatus, had been wounded in making the section of the prepuce; in a third, owing to 'œdema and difficulty of ascertaining where the glans was, amputation had been performed, and the end of the glans included.' The second variety of stricture was caused by the prepuce being divided too high up, or, what amounts to the same thing, being drawn down too much over the glans penis, before being included in the forceps for the purpose of making the necessary section. On bringing together the parts with sutures, the tension on them was so great as to cause ulceration, and to leave behind a broad cicatrix, capable of exercising a contractile pressure on the under surface of the urethra; sufficient to impede micturition and to cause other discomfort.'[19]

Dr. Hyde (*Boston Medical and Surgical Journal*, June 26, 1890) has seen disastrous results from circumcision; and Dr. Willard (in Keating's *Cyclopædia of the Diseases of Children*) says that, after circumcision, hardening of the glans occurs; and the evils of contracted meatus, balanitis, &c. follow, as pointed out by Otis, Mastin and others. So far, therefore, as the remote consequences of circumcision are concerned, there is strong evidence that the operation is by no means an unmixed blessing to its recipient.[20]

Turning to the more immediate effects and consequences, the italicised passages in Mr. Erichsen's elaborate description concur with the experience since cited of other writers, to show the need of considerable caution in the performance of this surgical procedure. Septic infection, hæmorrhage, and subsequent sloughing of the part have to be sedulously guarded against; and on the Continent, at least, the resources of modern antiseptic surgery have been specially invoked. Without careful ligature of the arteries, these may, we are told, give rise to troublesome and long unnoticed hæmorrhage when the patient is put back to bed. The examples above quoted, and the varying practice of different surgeons, show, moreover, that discrimination and judgment are essential as to the excision of either too much or too little of the foreskin; both of which events may be disadvantageous.

Mr. W. H. Jacobson (*Operations of Surgery*, 1889) says that after circumcision 'an adult should lie in bed for forty-eight hours, and keep on the sofa for a week, alternate stitches being removed at intervals. If he insist on getting about too early, he must run the risk of the parts remaining *long œdematous and tender*. And for this reason, with hospital patients, who have to come backwards and forwards, *early and complete healing is not to be expected*. (The italics are the present writer's.)

It may be reasonably assumed that no sane man, who possessed the advantages of a sound and entire prepuce, would willingly sacrifice it without just and sufficient cause being shown. And his natural repugnance to such a deprivation

---

[19] In the same work its author states that an unnatural smallness of the urethra is a not infrequent cause of incontinence of urine in children. In some cases therefore ascribed to congenital phimosis, may not the incontinence be merely a concomitant, and not an effect, of the latter condition?

[20] Dr. Keyes (*Diseases of Urinary Organs*, 1888) has been 'twice called upon to relieve by operation a phimosis resulting from a former operation.'

would probably be in no wise lessened by a perusal of the passage last cited. It would be without doubt in the highest degree edifying in the present connection, were the sensations of some educated adult of average sensitiveness, who had submitted to the operation, placed on record; together with a statement of the time which elapsed before perfect tolerance became established; and before the 'hard skinlike condition,' so much approved of by Mr. J. Hutchinson, and the other more or less enthusiastic advocates of circumcision, was satisfactorily attained. In the absence of such a delineation, however, we can only surmise the feelings of the patient; and conclude that, as with catheterisation, and other manipulations addressed to a delicate mucous membrane, they would in some instances be almost *nil*; but that in the man of highly sensitive organisation, they would amount to keen and long-protracted torture.

Infants of tender years must of necessity be classed in the latter of these two categories; in their case, there are also certain circumstances which tend to enhance the barbarity of the procedure; and largely to aggravate the suffering involved. Thus an American operator (at the association meeting of genito-urinary surgeons, reported in the *Boston Med. and Surg. Journal*, June 26, 1890) speaks of the difficulty of keeping children's knees out of the way after removal of the prepuce, and of the consequent torture to them. Even after healing, contact with flannel napkins, and other clothing, must long be very painful. There can be little doubt what would be the verdict—could they only give it utterance—upon the immediate results of the operation in question; returned by these inarticulate (if far from mute) victims of hygienic orthodoxy.[21]

[21] An objection to circumcision, of wholly sentimental character, yet not the less worthy of practical consideration, may, in addition to those set forth in the text, be here noted. The parents of any child, in whom the necessity of some remedial measure for congenital phimosis has become apparent, usually express considerable relief when told that it is not necessary to make the infant 'a little Jew.'

VI.

ABSENCE OF NECESSITY FOR CIRCUMCISION IN CASES OF CONGENITAL PHIMOSIS—THE RATIO-NAL TREATMENT OF THE LATTER.

From what has been already set forth, it is sufficiently evident that no male should be suffered to reach adult life with this congenital disability unrelieved; and that in the majority of instances radical treatment is requisite at a far earlier date. There can be no doubt that it is infinitely better for an infant to be subjected to circumcision, than to pass many months or years with the unpleasant or even dangerous symptoms previously detailed. The point now to be considered, therefore, is whether these symptoms can be obviated by any less heroic measure, and whether the suffering thus incurred is a matter of absolute necessity; whether, indeed, it is right and proper to subject the child to *mutilation* for the benevolent purpose indicated.

For by no less term can the procedure in question be characterised. It consists in the abstraction of a structure, not indeed of paramount importance to the organism, but obviously evolved by Nature for wise ends as a protective covering. Were there no necessity for its presence, it would not occur; and without overwhelming evidence that such mutilation is unavoidable and beneficial, it must be held ethically criminal thus to lay rough hands upon a perfectly normal organ.

As indicated above, congenital phimosis may be said in some slight degree to occur in every new-born male child. Two layers of muco-cutaneous membrane are developed in close contact, and are commonly agglutinated in a measure; but it is only when the separation is very incomplete that any defect producing consequences of importance is found. There is no deformity or deficiency of parts; and, except as a consequence of long-continued inflammation, no contraction occurs. What is commonly spoken of as 'a contracted prepuce' simply signifies the natural growth of the glans under a rigid envelope, primarily of normal proportions.

All, then, that is requisite to remedy this condition in the first instance, is the due separation of the two contiguous layers of muco-cutaneous membranes, which in the new-born may generally be effected with ease. As the infant grows, however, there is apt to supervene relative disparity of size; the tissues cannot be sufficiently expanded to allow of the ideal state of the organ—a prepuce movable freely and loosely upon its included glans—without some laceration. And, unless care be taken, the wounds in the parietal layer of muco-cutaneous membrane again quickly heal; the new cicatricial tissue undergoes, perhaps, a little real contraction; and matters remain as they were before. Hence, probably, the disfavour with which procedures, involving dilatation of the prepuce, seem to have been hitherto regarded by most surgeons.[22] Some amount of reunion between the two surfaces may also take place at the spots where the adhesions have been ruptured.

The principle to be aimed at, however, is simply the separation of two contiguous and adherent layers of mucous or muco-cutaneous membrane. Few medical men are probably aware of the natural distensibility of the parts; of the ease with which (when the patient is rendered passive and unconscious by means of an anæsthetic) the glans can be brought completely into view, and the prepuce perfectly retracted behind the corona. All that is then necessary is, by the use of emollients and by daily retraction for a very brief period, to prevent reunion of adhesions or of fissures in the muco-cutaneous membrane; until a sufficient degree of dilatation has been secured to preclude all fear of any future difficulty.

Certain precautions are, of course, necessary. The patient should be anæsthetised; the tissues involved are extremely sensitive, and the administration of ether (or of chloroform in the case of a young child), besides relaxing the parts, enables the measure to be carried out much more efficiently than would otherwise be the case. Although the necessary dilatation can usually be very speedily effected, it often takes some little time thoroughly to remove the adherent smegma, not seldom of gritty and calcareous consistence. This, besides being the longest, is the most painful part of the manipulation. The use of cocaine as a local anæsthetic for such a purpose, precluding the administration of ether or chloroform, is not to be recommended. The wide surface involved renders its influence incomplete; and it is of considerable advantage to have the patient, particularly when of tender years, oblivious to what is going on.[23]

If the distension be too timidly effected, so that the foreskin can be retracted over the glans only with difficulty; an equal difficulty will be found in pulling it forwards again, and temporary paraphimosis may result. Under anæsthesia, however, this cannot but prove transient; but if free dilatation be procured in the first instance, there is not the least fear of its occurrence at all.

On the other hand, care is requisite not to lacerate unnecessarily the delicate membrane; after which more or less inflammatory trouble supervenes, and the necessary daily retraction of the foreskin, to be subsequently insisted on, becomes difficult and painful. Should much œdema thus occur, it is best to discontinue for a few days the retraction, until the inflammation has subsided; substituting the daily injection with a syringe under the prepuce of warm carbolised oil, in such a manner that (the orifice being closed), the fluid is made to distend and 'balloon'

---

[22] For instance, Mr. Erichsen (*op. cit.*) dismisses the measure with the cursory allusion of a brief paragraph; against the long and elaborate account, previously detailed, of circumcision; it is not mentioned at all in the earlier editions of his work. Ashby and Wright speak of it with great disfavour. Mr. Jacobson (*Operations of Surgery*, 1890) does not introduce it at all; possibly because hardly worthy to be dignified by the title 'operation.'

[23] In adults, or in boys approaching manhood, gradual dilatation by the daily introduction of a sponge tent has been recommended. It might be resorted to in the case of an exceptionally timid and patient individual, but hardly for any other.

that envelope as much as possible.

The ideal dilatation-procedure is how to effect the maximum of dilatation with the minimum of laceration. In boys of seven or eight and upwards, it is often easy to stretch the parts sufficiently to allow of easy retraction and of free movement backwards and forwards without a single rent in the membrane, and without the loss of a single drop of blood. In younger children, however, this structure is necessarily much more delicate, and easily torn, especially if there be struggling. In the latter case complete anæsthesia, plenty of deliberation, and the use of not too large an instrument, are elements of importance.

The following is the usual method of performing this manipulation—'operation' is much too grave a word: The only instrument needed is an ordinary dressing-forceps of average size in the case of an adult or boy of age above indicated; proportionately smaller with young infants, in whom, indeed, a probe will sometimes effect all that is requisite.

> The patient being well anæsthetised, the surgeon, taking the organ in his left hand, retracts as far as possible the foreskin. With his right he introduces the closed dressing-forceps as far as it will enter; making sure, of course, that he has not passed it into the meatus. He then widely expands the two limbs of the handle, holding these apart for a few seconds. Complete retraction of the foreskin behind the corona glandis is then usually at once easy; adherent spots being separated with the thumb-nail. Should there be any difficulty the tissue is gradually peeled off by manipulation with the fingers; and the collections of inspissated smegma scraped off with the nail or with an ear-scoop. Finally, the operator pulls the prepuce backwards and forwards two or three times, making sure that it is perfectly loose; anoints the glans well with vaseline, and leaves it covered by the foreskin as in the normal state.

Subsequently, complete retraction is necessary on each of the first four or five days; after which it may be gradually intermitted, being subsequently resorted to only for purposes of cleanliness. The daily washing recommended by some American writers seems wholly unnecessary; and, as before remarked, the less tampering with these organs (except when absolutely unavoidable) the better. When free movement of the foreskin on the glans has been attained, together with healing of any excoriation or sore, there is no fear of subsequent contraction. Any seeming redundance of the prepuce is in no way detrimental; it should only serve to induce a more careful habit of cleanliness, and the habitual use of those ablutions to which every man naturally resorts upon attaining years of discretion.

Dilatation thus effected can at the least do no harm, and cannot possibly place the subject in a worse position than he was previously;—which the examples in previous chapters show to be far from the case, with the operation of circumcision. If carried out as here indicated, it will be found thoroughly effectual; the reasons why it appears to have failed in some hands apparently being: (*a*) neglect of after-treatment, and of care to retract the prepuce daily throughout the first few days; (*b*) insufficient dilatation at the time, so that retraction has never been perfectly easy; (*c*) avoidable and unnecessary laceration of the muco-cutaneous structures, followed by inflammatory mischief.[24]

The adoption of a special instrument for the above purpose has been advocated from time to time by several writers, who speak in glowing terms of the favourable results they have thus attained. A rather formidable-looking one, used by Nélaton, is depicted in the *Gazette des Hôpitaux*, 31, 1868; this has three blades at right angles to the stem, and is somewhat on the model of an ordinary urethral dilator. Several successful cases are described, with one of failure. In the latter, a youth of seventeen, incision had to be resorted to, as the prepuce could not be stretched sufficiently with the instrument; and in this there was doubtless true contraction, probably as a result of venereal infection.

In the *Dublin Quarterly Journal*, No. xlviii. p. 482, Dr. Cruise, of Dublin, figures a somewhat analogous instrument with two blades, and speaks of numerous cases ('in which with due care the result has been perfect') in his own hands and in those of his friends. He, however, kept the foreskin subsequently retracted for twenty-four to forty-eight hours, a proceeding which entails upon the patient very considerable discomfort, and is unnecessary. Dr. Hayes Agnew (*Principles of Surgery*) figures a special 'phimosis-forceps,' which appears in no essential particular to differ from ordinary dressing-forceps; the only noticeable peculiarity being that the blades are a little longer than usual. Levis's dilatation-instrument, described in Keating's *Cyclopædia*, vol. iii. p. 643, is worked by screw-power, and is stated to be 'very effective;' it resembles an ordinary pair of dissecting-forceps, with a screw placed close to the handle, which effects separation of the two blades. This is, no doubt, satisfactory in its results, but seems to be unnecessarily severe for the purpose to which it is applied; in which very little force is usually needed, or, indeed, is desirable, for obvious reasons. Mr. R. W. Parker's dilatation-instrument has been referred to on the previous page; and there are doubtless many others.

Dr. F. H. Stuart, of Brooklyn (*Medical Record*, December 4, 1886), in advocating a manipulation very similar to the one here described (he introduces first a probe to break down adhesions, then the dressing-forceps, turning the latter round); comes to the conclusion that 'the number of cases which really require circumcision is extremely small.' And it may be generally remarked that no one who has really tried the dilatation plan with due care and without prejudice, appears to have subsequently relinquished it; or to have been otherwise than highly satisfied with its effects, whatever the precise method adopted. Those surgeons who speak of having seen unsatisfactory results generally convey the idea that these have taken place in other hands; and have never, in any publication seen by the present writer, condescended to details.[25]

[24] Mr. R. W. Parker (*Brit. Med. Journal*, July 19, 1879) recommends gradual dilatation with a special screw-forceps, which he has used in a considerable number of cases at the Children's Hospital, 'always with good results.'

[25] In the paper above quoted, by Dr. Cruise, of Dublin (1868), that surgeon speaks of Dr. Hutton having used dressing-forceps for the cure of phimosis fifteen years previously. Very probably the adoption of that instrument for the same purpose would be found on in-

To the case of boys past the early years of childhood, and still more to that of adults, the arguments in favour of the substitution of a simple dilatation-process for the unnecessarily severe operation of circumcision, apply with redoubled force. As in these no symptoms directing attention to the phimosis have previously existed for any length of time, it may be taken at once for granted that, however tight the so-called 'contraction' may seem on inspection, the condition is present in only a minor degree; that under an anæsthetic the adhesions will yield to very slight force, and satisfactory retraction, with subsequent free mobility, be procured without the slightest difficulty. With adults, moreover, the avoidance of any need for confinement to bed, of even to the house, is an important consideration. In such the tissues are necessarily more elastic and less fragile than in young infants; there is much less prospect of laceration, with consequent tenderness and swelling.

An operation for the relief of congenital phimosis advocated by Mr. Furneaux Jordan (*British Medical Journal*, May 2, 1863) may be here alluded to.

> Mr. Jordan passes one blade of a small round-pointed scissors (Critchett's strabismus-scissors answer well) through the orifice; skin and mucous membrane are divided to the length of a quarter of an inch on one side, the same being repeated on the other. The prepuce is now retracted as far as possible; this exposes more lining membrane between the lips of the wound, and this again is divided by a second incision on each side. The operation is now complete, and the foreskin may easily be retracted.

> The incisions which were made in the long axis of the penis after retraction become linear in a vertical direction, and almost imperceptible in the circular folds of retracted foreskin. In the after-treatment the prepuce should be kept back, or frequently retracted. In children retraction once daily for a week or ten days, till the wounds have healed, is quite sufficient. The extent of the incisions should, of course, be a little less in children, a little greater in the adult.

The present writer has seen this operation performed in one instance, and the after-results were in the highest degree satisfactory. As contrasted with circumcision, the procedure merits warm commendation; preserving the useful foreskin, and followed by a much more speedy recovery than may be expected from the former. For the lacerations which may result from forcible dilatation, small nicks with a pair of scissors are substituted. The only objection is that even this operation, trivial as it appears, is seldom necessary; and that sufficient distension of the foreskin may often be procured without any breach of surface whatever. Moreover, some confinement to bed or to the sofa is subsequently requisite; whereas, after the effects of the anæsthetic have passed off, the patient, young or old, whose foreskin has been dilated, can behave exactly as usual.[26]

quiry to date back still further; and no pretension of originality can be here put forth for the advocacy of a simple common-sense practice, which must have been repeatedly resorted to by many practitioners of the past.

[26] M. Faure has also described a somewhat analogous 'nicking' operation.

Mr. Jordan's operation is, however, a very useful corollary to the dilatation-method in the chronic phimosis (often associated with gout) of men in advanced life; when the parts are usually in a very gristly condition; and when, if it be found impossible to procure retraction by stretching, the contracted tissues may be advantageously nicked with scissors in the mode here indicated.

VII.

SUMMARY.

I. Circumcision as a sacrificial rite has been practised by very numerous races of diverse origin, and dates from an extremely remote antiquity; probably from the Stone Age, as suggested by the internal evidence of Biblical records.

II. This fact, together with that of its application by many tribes to the persons of female children, deprives the religious ceremony of any title to the hygienic character and purpose, which have been frequently attributed to it.

III. The surgical operation of circumcision, especially where infants are concerned, has therefore to be discussed solely on its own merits, wholly apart from any theory of Divine intentions, based upon theological considerations. It appears to be erroneous *in principle*.

IV. It consists in a *mutilation*; in the removal of a perfectly normal structure, with which, for patent physiological reasons, every male child is endowed by nature. The morality of such a practice, without grave necessity, is open to question.

V. Unless as the result of subsequent disease, no deformity, and indeed no actual abnormality, exist as factors productive of the condition designated 'Congenital Phimosis.' Almost every male child suffers at birth from some degree of the same phenomenon—the imperfect separation of two muco-cutaneous surfaces, developed in contiguity.[27]

VI. Symptoms ascribed to a 'contracted prepuce' are due to natural growth of the glans penis, when this physiological separation is very incomplete, and when, therefore, a rigid constricting envelope prevents development. *No true contraction* exists, except as the result of superadded inflammation; and is rarely of much importance, unless an element of contagion has been introduced.

VII. The rational treatment of congenital phimosis primarily consists in the efficient execution of the process originally intended by nature, but imperfectly carried out. And, secondarily, in precautions to ensure the permanently free mobility of the prepuce upon the glans penis.

VIII. Such complete separation of the two contiguous layers of membrane may almost invariably be effected by very simple means; and, with some slight attention to after-treatment, will permanently secure all that is desired, without risk

---

[27] The word 'adhesion' in the previous pages is employed solely as a term of convenience, to denote this imperfect separation, and does not imply any analogy to inflammatory processes.

and without even transient disability.

IX. The treatment of congenital phimosis by dilatation is the common-sense remedy for this condition. It has been carried out by many practitioners with different instruments and variations of detail; and all who have thus attempted it with ordinary care (including the present writer) seem eminently satisfied with the results.[28]

X. When diseased processes co-exist with congenital phimosis, the case must necessarily be treated on its own merits. Simple dilatation, even if practicable, is not always sufficient, but should be combined with incisions of as limited a nature as possible. Mr. Furneaux Jordan's operation is then useful.

XI. In the event of disease, the operation of circumcision is not devoid of risk, and should be reserved as far as possible for extreme cases, in which removal of the whole prepuce is obviously a matter of necessity.[29]

XII. In healthy children the operation seems to be rarely fatal in this country. Many cases of death directly traceable to circumcision have, however, been reported on the Continent.

XIII. The immediate effects of circumcision, especially when performed on young infants, involve considerable and protracted suffering.

XIV. The most conspicuous *remote* result is that of an extremely contracted *meatus urinarius*, as the consequence of subsequent inflammatory processes, due to the exposure and continual friction of the unprotected glans.

XV. The compulsory enforcement of local cleanliness procured by circumcision seems hardly a sufficient argument for the general adoption of the practice by peoples not utterly indifferent to all laws of hygiene; and has little weight even in individual cases.

XVI. The superior chastity and purity of mind and body supposed to be procured for its recipients by ritual circumcision, lie open to very considerable question, in the face of abundant well-known facts.

XVII. The advantage of circumcision in obviating future venereal contagion is restricted by its principal advocate to one form (albeit the most important) of such disease. Even in this limited field the facts adduced appear open to dispute, and greatly to need confirmation by independent observers.

XVIII. In the hands of careless or inexperienced operators the surgical operation of circumcision has been followed by the most disastrous permanent consequences.

---

[28] The writer first drew attention to the advantages of this method of treatment in the *British Medical Journal*, Nov. 15, 1874. Having instituted a tolerably extensive search through the medical literature of the preceding three or four decades, he is unable to find any account of a case in which the procedure failed to effect a permanent cure, unless there had existed previous disease.

[29] A fatal case, after circumcision for gonorrhœal inflammation, in a youth of 17, is reported in the *Lancet*, Feb. 25, 1882. Death took place on the eighth day apparently from septicæmic pneumonia.

XIX. In face of the facts here set forth, it is NOT advisable to apply the operation of circumcision, as a remedy for congenital phimosis, to Christian infants; much less to extend this, as a routine custom, to the whole male population.

BIBLIOGRAPHY.

PUBLISHED WORKS.

I.—MEDICAL.

Erichsen's *Surgery*, Ninth Edition; Holmes's *System of Surgery*, Third Edition; Maunder's *Operative Surgery*; Joseph Bell's *Manual of Surgical Operations*; Jacobson's *Operations of Surgery*; Reginald Harrison's *Diseases of Urinary Organs*, Third Edition; Keyes's *Diseases of Urinary Organs*; Keating's *Cyclopædia of the Diseases of Children*; Ashby and Wright's *Diseases of Children*; Jaffé's *Die rituelle Circumcision im Lichte der antiseptischen Chirurgie*; Asher's *The Jewish Rite of Circumcision*; Wunderbar's *Biblisch-Talmudische Medicin*; Gideon Bircher's *Die Beschneidung der Israeliten*; Dr. Hayes Agnew's *Principles of Surgery*; Sayre's *Orthopædic Surgery*; Hilton's *Rest and Pain*; *International Encyclopædia of Surgery*, 1886; *Guy's Hospital Reports*; *American Journal of Syphilis and Dermatology*, October 1872; Walsham's *Theory and Practice of Surgery*, &c. &c.

II.—HISTORICAL AND MISCELLANEOUS.

The Testaments, Old and New; *The Talmud*; *Maimonides on Circumcision*; Tylor's *Primitive Culture*; Moncure Conway's *Demonology and Devil Lore*; Keil's *Biblical Archæology*; Smith's *Dictionary of the Bible*; Calmet, *Dictionary of the Bible, Encyclopædia Americana, Encyclopædia Britannica*; Howard, *Royal Encyclopædia*; *Penny Cyclopædia*; *Chambers's Encyclopædia*; *Encyclopædia Metropolitana*; Winer's *Realwörth*; Brewster, *Edinburgh Encyclopædia*; *English Cyclopædia*; Wilkes's *Encyclopædia Londinensis*; *Globe Encyclopædia*, &c.

PERIODICALS.

The Lancet, British Medical Journal, Medical Times and Gazette, Medical Record, Dublin Journal, Boston Medical and Surgical Journal, Chicago Medical Standard, Gazette des Hôpitaux, Allgemeine Wiener Med. Zeitung, Wiener Med. Presse, &c.

Lector House believes that a society develops through a two-fold approach of continuous learning and adaptation, which is derived from the study of classic literary works spread across the historic timeline of literature records. Therefore, we aim at reviving, repairing and redeveloping all those inaccessible or damaged but historically as well as culturally important literature across subjects so that the future generations may have an opportunity to study and learn from past works to embark upon a journey of creating a better future.

This book is a result of an effort made by Lector House towards making a contribution to the preservation and repair of original ancient works which might hold historical significance to the approach of continuous learning across subjects.

HAPPY READING & LEARNING!

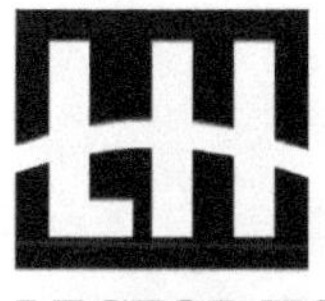

LECTOR HOUSE LLP
E-MAIL: lectorpublishing@gmail.com

www.ingramcontent.com/pod-product-compliance
Lightning Source LLC
Chambersburg PA
CBHW051408130726
47987CB00007B/2900